CANCER AGAIN?!

A Personal Journey of Hope and Inspiration

CANCER AGAIN?!

A Personal Journey of Hope and Inspiration

Sandy Foreman

> A percentage of the profits from the sale of the book will be donated to cancer research.

Russ Ranch Productions
Woodacre, California

CANCER AGAIN?! by Sandy Foreman

Russ Ranch Productions
Post Office Box 517
Woodacre, CA 94973-0517 U.S.A.

All rights reserved. No part of this book may be reproduced or transmitted in any form or by any means, electronic or mechanical, including photocopying, recording or by any information storage and retrieval system without the written permission from author, except for the inclusion of brief quotations in a review.

Unattributed quotations are by Sandy Foreman.

Copyright © 2014 by Sandy Foreman.

Illustrations by Cristina Soto, Sandy Foreman

ISBN 978-0-9908627-0-3

First Edition 2014

This book is dedicated to all cancer survivors. I consider you all to be my brothers and sisters. We are warriors, and, yes, we are special.

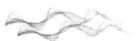

Contents

Forward ix

Acknowledgements xiii

About the Author xv

Introduction 1

Quality of Life 3

Being Aware 9

Family and Friends 13

Life Values 19

Your Doctor and Oncology Staff 25

We're All Different 31

Idle Time 35

Humility 39

Hair or No Hair 43

Comfort 49

Inner Spirit 53

Support 59

Take Time for Yourself 63

Let's Stay Positive 67

Inspiration 71

The Human Body 75

Eat Well and Live Well 81

Love Yourself 85

Celebrate Life 91

Afterword 95

Forward

Can you think of someone whose influence changed the course of your life? Sandy Foreman was that person for me. In 1991, I met her at Unity Center in Walnut Creek, California. When I walked into Unity Center, I was a lost soul with no direction in my life. At the time, I worked at a dead-end sales job where I was bored and unfulfilled. I had no ambition or plans for my future.

Unity is a spiritual organization that teaches us how to: connect with the presence of God within, positively change our thinking, and live happy and prosperous lives.

I met Sandy as I was standing on the patio one Sunday at Unity Center. She was the Youth Education Director. When I told Sandy that I was a certificated teacher, she instantly encouraged me to teach Sunday School. I accepted Sandy's offer, and my spiritual journey began.

Being new to Unity, I needed to learn Unity principles. It was the high school Sunday School students that taught me the spiritual principles that I have grown to love and teach. It was Sandy Foreman who taught me to find my inner strength and to follow the desires of my heart. Sandy encouraged me to run for the Board of Trustees at Unity Center. She encouraged me to take Unity Classes to deepen my knowledge and skills. Sandy encouraged me to go to ministerial school to become a Unity Minister.

I worked with Sandy again at the Unity Church of Maui. While there, I saw her face her second bout with cancer. She never let it get her down. She was always positive and believed that she would recover. She taped positive affirmations on the screen of her computer monitor. Throughout her journey with cancer she continued to do her job with love and passion.

Sandy is an incredible example of strength, faith and love. She showed strength by practicing the spiritual principles that she believed in. She practiced faith by knowing that God was expressing perfectly through her no matter what was happening with her body. She practiced love by loving herself and everyone in her life.

Sandy has had a positive and powerful effect on my life. She encouraged me to discover who

Forward

I am and to live up to my highest possibility. I know that her book will empower you to discover your truth and to follow your dreams.

Sandy, I am eternally grateful for all that you have helped me to discover about myself. You are truly a perfect expression of God.

Love and Blessings,
Reverend Blaine Tinsley

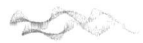

Acknowledgments

My friends and family have supported me as I've put my feelings down on paper.

I want to thank my Maui Soul Sisters group– you've always been there for me with your genuine encouragement. Thanks to Joanne Laucher, Laurie Mann, Edie Van Hoose, Suzanne Douglas, Jodie Easler, Cynthia Thiede, and Carole Cote'.

Special gratitude goes to my loving husband, Charlie. Thank you for being my rock and number one care and love giver.

Heaps of thanks to my son, David Russ, for his expert job of layout, editing and publication– you've been superb.

More thanks to my 13-year-old granddaughter, Cristina Soto, for her original, creative illustrations that lent a little whimsy to a serious topic.

Special thanks to my 10-year-old grandson, Joshua Soto, for allowing me to use his thought

Acknowledgments

enhancing story of Chief Clawing Bear. The story gives us a lesson on life values.

It has been a marvelous adventure for me and you have all been there with me every step of the way. Thank you.

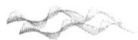

About the Author

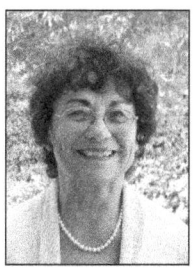

Sandy Foreman is a two-time cancer survivor. She was diagnosed with breast cancer in 2005, then uterine cancer in 2012. She beat them both, but her mother was not so lucky and died of cancer at the age of 53 in 1971.

Sandy was born in San Francisco in 1942. At age 12 she moved to Sunnyvale, California and attended Benner Middle School and graduated from Fremont Union High School in 1960. She now resides in Walnut Creek, California.

Sandy has been married to Charlie for over 30 years who has been loving and supportive for all these years.

Participating in Relay For Life in Maui and the Susan G. Komen San Francisco Walk, Sandy has helped raise funds for cancer research. Also, a portion of the proceeds from the sale of this book will be donated to cancer research. She has seen the many advances that cancer research has made over the years and gives thanks to those who have also donated to the search for a cure for cancer.

Introduction

After having survived cancer twice, my heart told me to share my experience with others who might find my story . . .

Inspiring
Heartwarming
Helpful
Genuine, Heartfelt
Encouraging
Sincere

My hope is that **"Cancer Again?!"** will be the positive message that with love, support, and positive thinking we will again, live healthy, prosperous and happy lives.

I have a deep appreciation for cancer research. I've seen strides from when my mother died of cancer in 1971, to my two encounters with cancer, along with many of my friends and family members who have also experienced the cancer challenge. I want to thank the many cancer research programs by giving a percentage of the profits from this book to them, with my deepest gratitude.

Cancer Again?!

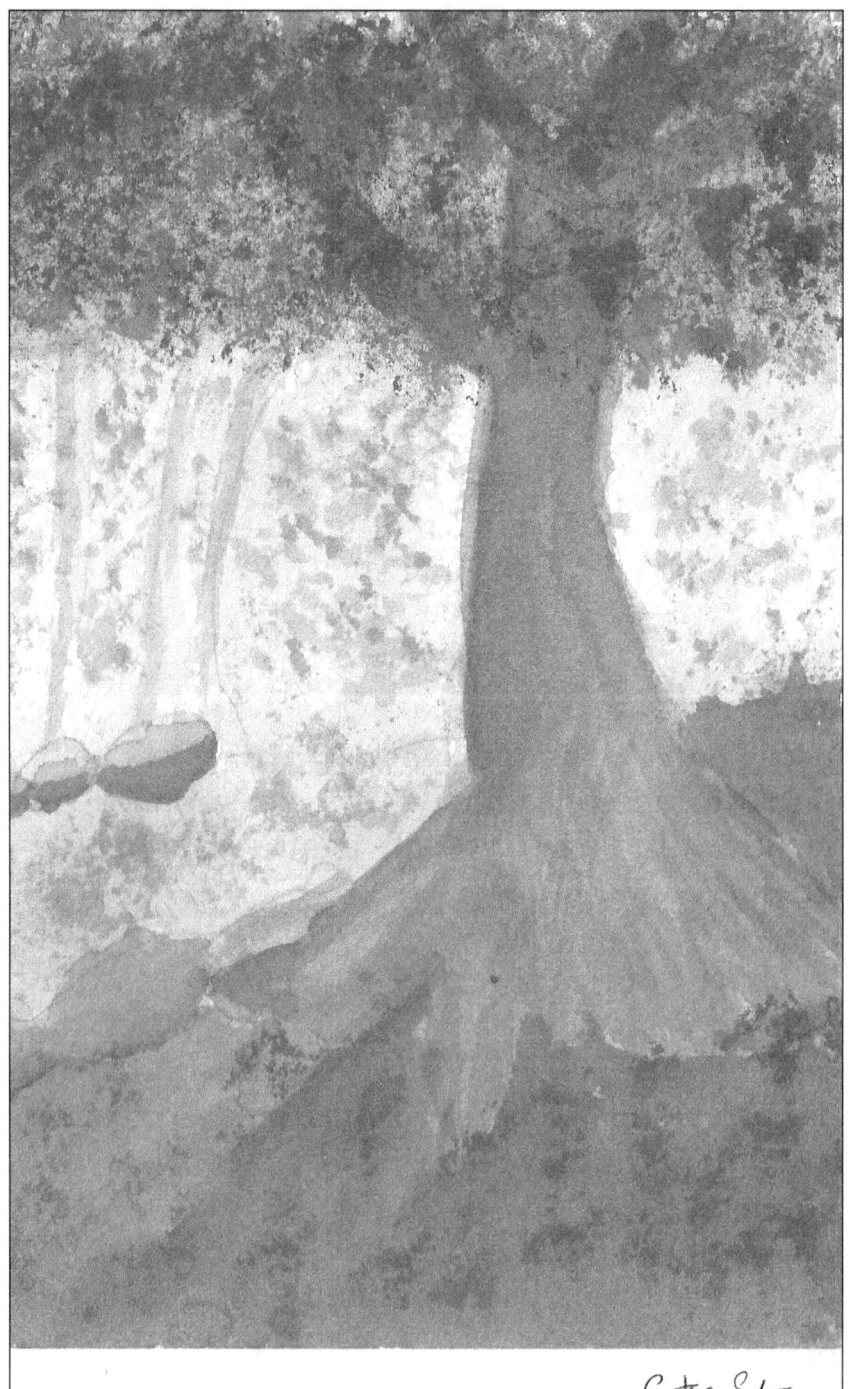

Quality of Life

Once your diagnosis has set in you may ask yourself, "What will be my quality of life now that I have this realization–I have cancer!" From my experience, your quality of life will be however you choose it to be. You can think of yourself as less than the person you were before your diagnosis or you can choose to believe here's an obstacle I will overcome.

If you're having to go through chemotherapy, you'll probably lose your hair. Oh, no! But how about choosing to think differently than 'Oh, no!'. Go online and check out the cute hats, scarves and wigs you have to choose from. You can be downright stylish! Play with it, how about a pink wig??? Why not? Mix your scarves with your hats or twist them around turban style. Women wore them in a most stylish fashion in the 40's–bring back the drama. Feeling good about yourself will help determine your quality of life.

Thinking is believing. Some mornings you will wake up and feel awful; other days you'll feel okay. Regardless of how your mind is telling you how you feel, start by counting your blessings. Number one, you woke up. "Thank you, God, for giving me one more glorious day on earth." If you can go outside, take a short walk and appreciate nature. Take in a deep breath and say, "Thanks". If you cannot go outside, walk around your living space and admire some of your precious belongings. Have a sacred alter with certain items placed on it that give you peace and contentment. Always live in gratitude for your quality of life.

Call a friend or family member and share your positive outlook. Just doing that will give them pleasure.

Cancer is only a bleep in the radar, it's not your whole life; don't give it power over you!

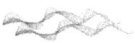

Affirmation: *"I am healthy, well and wholesome."*

Quote: *"As the clouds roll by, you'll be happy to see the sun."*

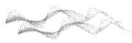

Scripture: *Ask and it shall be given to you, seek and ye shall find, knock and it shall be opened unto you.*
Matthew 7:7

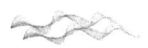

My Space For Thoughts, Reminders, Aha's

This space is for you to give gratitude, vent annoyances, remark on profound realizations, give appreciation to yourself, etc. Please use this area for whatever thoughts and feelings give you pleasure.

<u>Be sure to date each entry</u>. I find it fun to look back at things I've written months or years ago and think, "I said what??? When was that???"

_____

_____

_____

_____

_____

_____

_____

_____

_____

Quality of Life

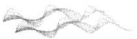

"Sandy's 'can do' attitude truly kicked into high-gear when she received the diagnosis. She knew without a doubt she would win! Chemotherapy, radiation, she approached it like "I can do this and not even miss a day of work, piece of cake." Her courage and optimism truly amazed and inspired me. I love her and am proud to have her as my friend."

Joanne Laucher

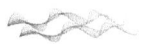

Cancer Again?!

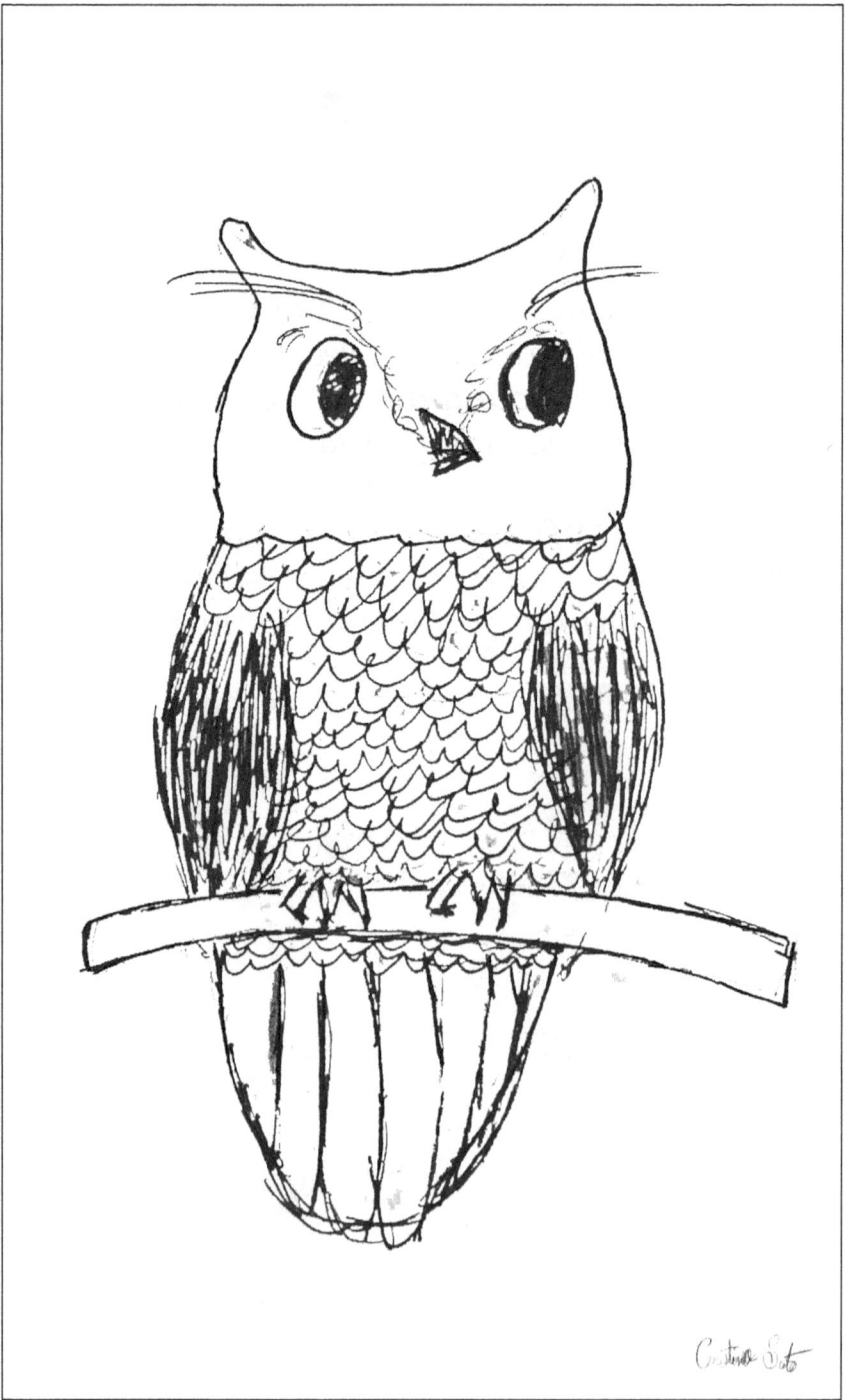

Being Aware

Early detection, early detection, early detection. I can't say it enough. Please don't ignore your body, it's the only one you've got. I've always been faithful with getting my mammograms regularly and as soon as something suspicious was spotted on the mammogram I was recommended to have a sonogram. From the sonagram I was advised that the doctors needed to take a biopsy. Surgery was the next step; cancer was found and chemotherapy and radiation treatments were started. In addition to having mammograms, please also do your breasts self-exams once a month. If you do them regularly you'll be more likely to notice any unusual changes.

Seven years later I noticed spotting from the uterus area; I went directly to my gynecologist. This time the diagnosis was cancer of the endometrial, adenocarcinoma.

The uterine cancer was diagnosed in February and my hysterectomy was performed in April. Again, I had chemotherapy, followed by radiation. This all worked well for me. You may decide to do alternative medicine and that is perfectly fine if you are totally comfortable with it. I followed the conventional medical methods because I felt after years and years of medical research this was the sure way to get me through this crisis. So far, so good.

My point is, please don't ignore signs alerting you that something in your body is wanting your attention. Act on it right now! Early detection is crucial.

Affirmation: *"I am proactive with my health."*

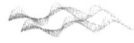

Quote: *"It's your story, be the hero."*

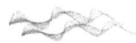

Scipture: *Take heed unto thyself, and unto the doctrine; continue in them: for in doing this thou shalt both save thyself, and them that hear thee.*

1 Timothy 4:16

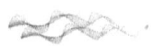

My Space For Thoughts, Reminders, Aha's

This space is for you to give gratitude, vent annoyances, remark on profound realizations, give appreciation to yourself, etc. Please use this area for whatever thoughts and feelings give you pleasure.

<u>Be sure to date each entry</u>. I find it fun to look back at things I've written months or years ago and think, "I said what??? When was that???"

_____

_____

_____

_____

_____

_____

_____

_____

_____

Cancer Again?!

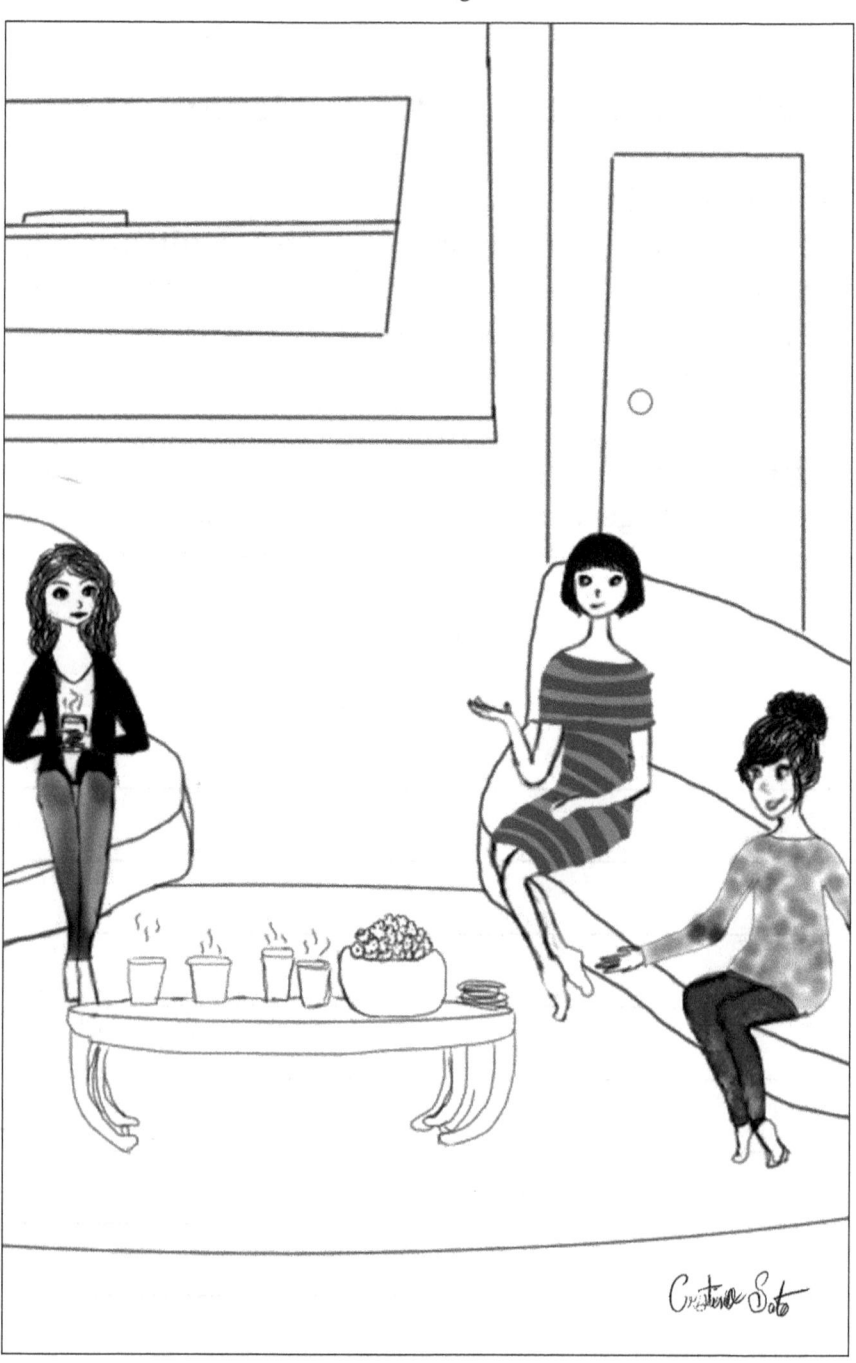

Family and Friends

It is a very delicate thing how we tell our family and friends that we've been diagnosed with cancer. I am lucky enough to have a loving husband who has been with me every step of this journey. He was with me when I first got the confirmation from the oncologist.

People react differently to the word cancer; so it is important to be honest about how you feel. Family and friends may feel scared, or at a loss for how to relate to you. It's all natural.

My grown son said he felt helpless; not knowing how to support me. My grown daughter said her first thought was to come and stay with me, but we lived 2500 miles apart and she had a family to care for.

Luckily I am a member of a very caring women's group. They were very loving and optimistic. They wanted to help in any way they could. When I reached the radiation stage, some of my 'soul sisters' wanted to drive me to my appointments which was a 40-minute drive each way; I could have driven myself–at that point I felt fine, but I knew they were offering me a gift. It was important to accept those gifts and allow them to drive me. It made them feel they were contributing to my well-being. I very much appreciated that and welcomed their companionship on the long ride. A lot of times it's stressful for your friends and family because they really want to help but are not sure how to do it. Please allow family and friends to help you, it's a gift both for you and for them.

You'll make new friends on the journey. You'll become a part of the sisterhood of cancer. You'll be amazed at how many acquaintances you already know who have also been faced with the cancer challenge. Once they know what you are going through, they will come forward and share their stories. All of a sudden, you will have a true bond with these people who before had been mere acquaintances. They will always be there to support you. So, please don't suffer in silence; we need all the support we can get at this time on our human path.

Also, you'll make friends with your medical caregivers. If you experience chemotherapy, you'll sit for many hours with these folks and they will become more that caregivers to you– they will become your friends.

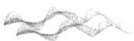

Affirmation: *"I have many loving friends."*

Quote: *"Express to your family and friends how happy you are to have them in your life."*

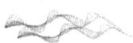

Scripture: *Faithful friends are beyond price; no amount can balance their worth.*

                                        Sirach 6:15

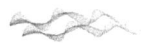

My Space For Thoughts, Reminders, Aha's

This space is for you to give gratitude, vent annoyances, remark on profound realizations, give appreciation to yourself, etc. Please use this area for whatever thoughts and feelings give you pleasure.

<u>Be sure to date each entry</u>. I find it fun to look back at things I've written months or years ago and think, "I said what??? When was that???"

_____

_____

_____

_____

_____

_____

_____

_____

_____

Family and Friends

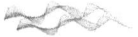

"*I found Sandy to be strong and brave through her cancer experiences. Never complaining or wanting a 'pity party'.*"

Cynthia Thiede

Cancer Again?!

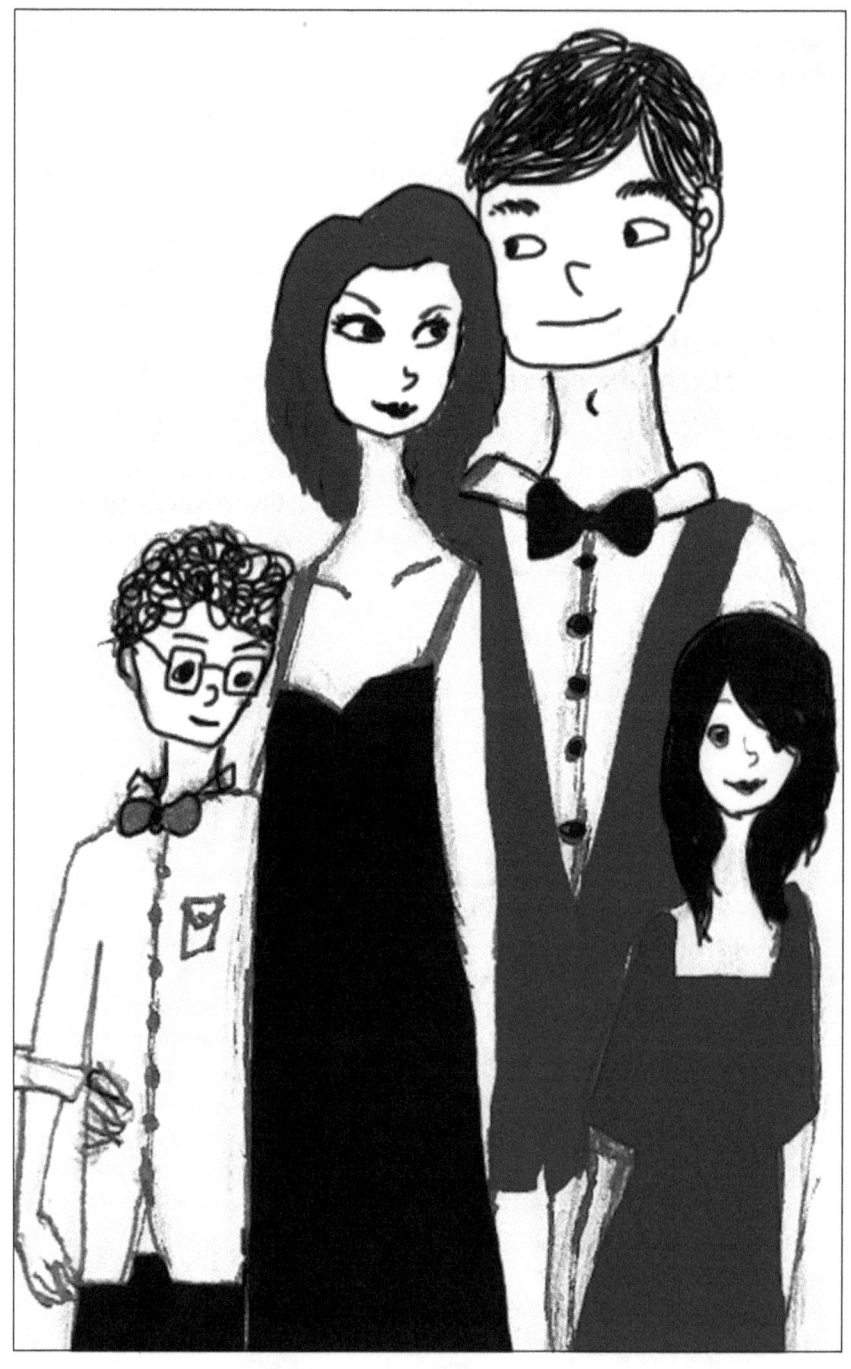

Life Values

Now is a good time to take an inventory of your life values. You might notice that your life values changed from the day before you were told you have cancer to the day after you were told you have cancer. What do you think?

Before I was diagnosed with cancer my life values would be to be wealthy, to be able to travel anywhere any time, to have a successful career, have nice clothes and nice cars, etc. All material things. But after hearing the words, "you have cancer" my values changed quite a bit.

God became my first life value. I remember going straight to prayer. "Oh, God, please help me through this health challenge." Not that I wasn't spiritual before, but after the diagnosis prayers were always on my lips.

So, this is a good time to take stock of your life values. Take time to write them out. Put your values in categories and prioritize them. Such as: your spirituality, your family, your friends, your pets, giving gratitude, being honest and trustworthy with yourself and others. Is good communication important to you? Add it to your list.

Be thoughtful about this exercise. It could lead to a more joyful life for you and those around you.

This is your life. You create how good or not so good it is through your life values.

If you are comfortable with sharing these thoughts with others, invite a friend in for tea and have a nice one-on-one conversation. Saying the words will imprint them on your soul and help to guide you forward.

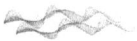

Affirmation: *"I am aware of my life values and live them daily."*

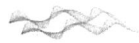

Quote: *"Be careful what you ask for, you just might get it."*

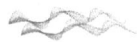

Scripture: *. . . These who do not have the law are a law to themselves. They show that the work of the law is written in their hearts, as their conscience bears witness and their conflicting thoughts accuse or else defend them.*
Romans 2:14-16

My Space For Thoughts, Reminders, Aha's

This space is for you to give gratitude, vent annoyances, remark on profound realizations, give appreciation to yourself, etc. Please use this area for whatever thoughts and feelings give you pleasure.

Be sure to date each entry. I find it fun to look back at things I've written months or years ago and think, "I said what??? When was that???"

_____

_____

_____

_____

_____

_____

_____

_____

_____

_____

Cancer Again?!

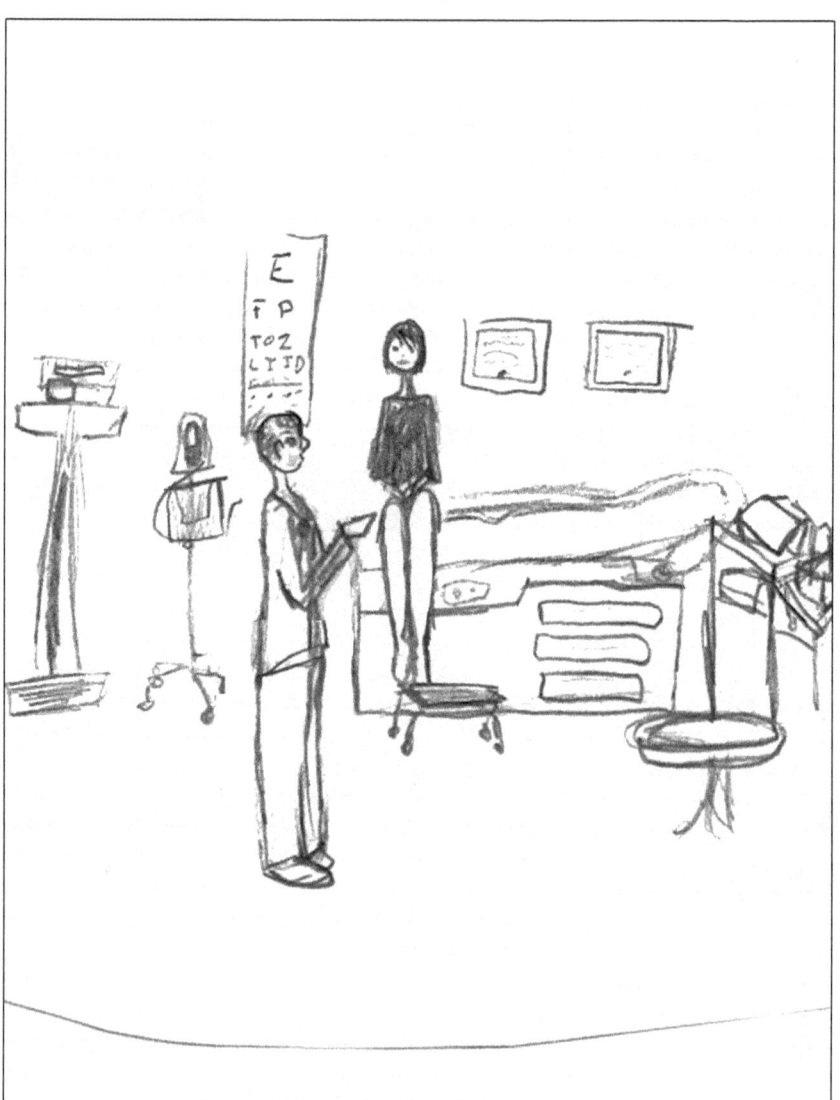

Your Doctor and Oncology Staff

It is important that you are comfortable with your oncologist. You will be seeing this person on a regular basis for a long while; therefore, you will need to be open to listening to the doctor and his staff. They are the experts.

Not that I would wish this on any of you, but when I returned seven years later to have chemo and radiation treatments again, my same oncologist nurse was there and greeted me with open arms. She was happy to see me but, of course, not under those conditions. Also, the two radiation technicians were both still there, and they remembered me. This helped me just knowing I was in the hands of good, caring friends.

Here are a few questions you might consider asking:

"What are my treatment options?"

"Why are you recommending this treatment plan?"

"What are clinical trials? Would you recommend one to me? Why or why not?"

"What are the side-effects of this treatment?"

"Will I be able to go to work?"

"Where can I find a cancer support group?"

"Who will be responsible for my follow-up care after my treatment?"

I'm sure you'll have more questions, write them down.

It is important to take time to talk openly and honestly with your doctor; it will help you to gain trust and confidence in him/her.

Find out as much as you can about the type of cancer you have. Here are a few internet sites to explore: www.cancercare.org, www.komen.org, www.cancer.org, www.cancer.gov.

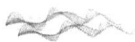

Affirmation: *"I have the strength to be whole and well."*

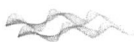

Quote: *"We don't have to fight cancer alone."*

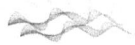

Scripture: *You are my refuge and my shield; I put my hope in your word.*
Psalms 119:114

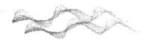

My Space For Thoughts, Reminders, Aha's

This space is for you to give gratitude, vent annoyances, remark on profound realizations, give appreciation to yourself, etc. Please use this area for whatever thoughts and feelings give you pleasure.

<u>Be sure to date each entry</u>. I find it fun to look back at things I've written months or years ago and think, "I said what??? When was that???"

_____

_____

_____

_____

_____

_____

_____

_____

_____

"Be grateful for whoever comes, because each has been sent as a guide from beyond."

Rumi

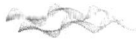

Cancer Again?!

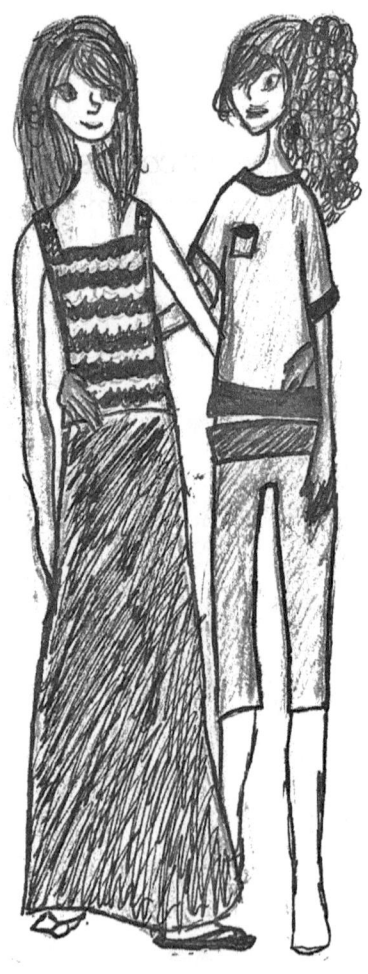

We're All Different,
Yet We're All The Same

When I was first diagnosed with cancer, it felt like I was the only one on earth who ever had cancer. I was self-absorbed. It was, "All about me!" As I got used to the idea, I knew I was going to be fine. Modern research had made gigantic strides toward the cure of cancer since my mother died of cancer in 1971. Therefore, the early detection of my breast cancer was a blessing and I just needed to follow the treatments that the oncologist set forth for me.

While sitting in the waiting room for my radiation treatment, the lady next to me started a conversation and as we discussed our different cancers we realized how courageous we both were. And, how connected we both were. Yes, we are sisters and a part of a huge family of cancer survivors. How wonderful!

You may not follow the conventional medical cancer treatments; you may opt to follow an alternative path, and that's okay. That's your choice and it will be the right one for you. Just know we're all here to support you.

What you may be going through now, may at sometime in the future be helpful information for someone else. Hopefully that gives you strength knowing at some point you may be of support to a friend or a new acquaintance.

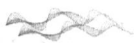

Affirmation: *"I am here to be an inspiration to others."*

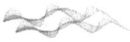

Quote: *"Once the treatments are over, you'll be proud to say, 'I DID IT!'"*

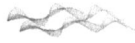

Scripture: *If all were a single member, where would the body be? As it is, there are many parts, yet one body.*
1 Corinthians 12:19-20

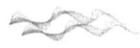

My Space For Thoughts, Reminders, Aha's

This space is for you to give gratitude, vent annoyances, remark on profound realizations, give appreciation to yourself, etc. Please use this area for whatever thoughts and feelings give you pleasure.

<u>Be sure to date each entry</u>. I find it fun to look back at things I've written months or years ago and think, "I said what??? When was that???"

_____

_____

_____

_____

_____

_____

_____

_____

_____

Cancer Again?!

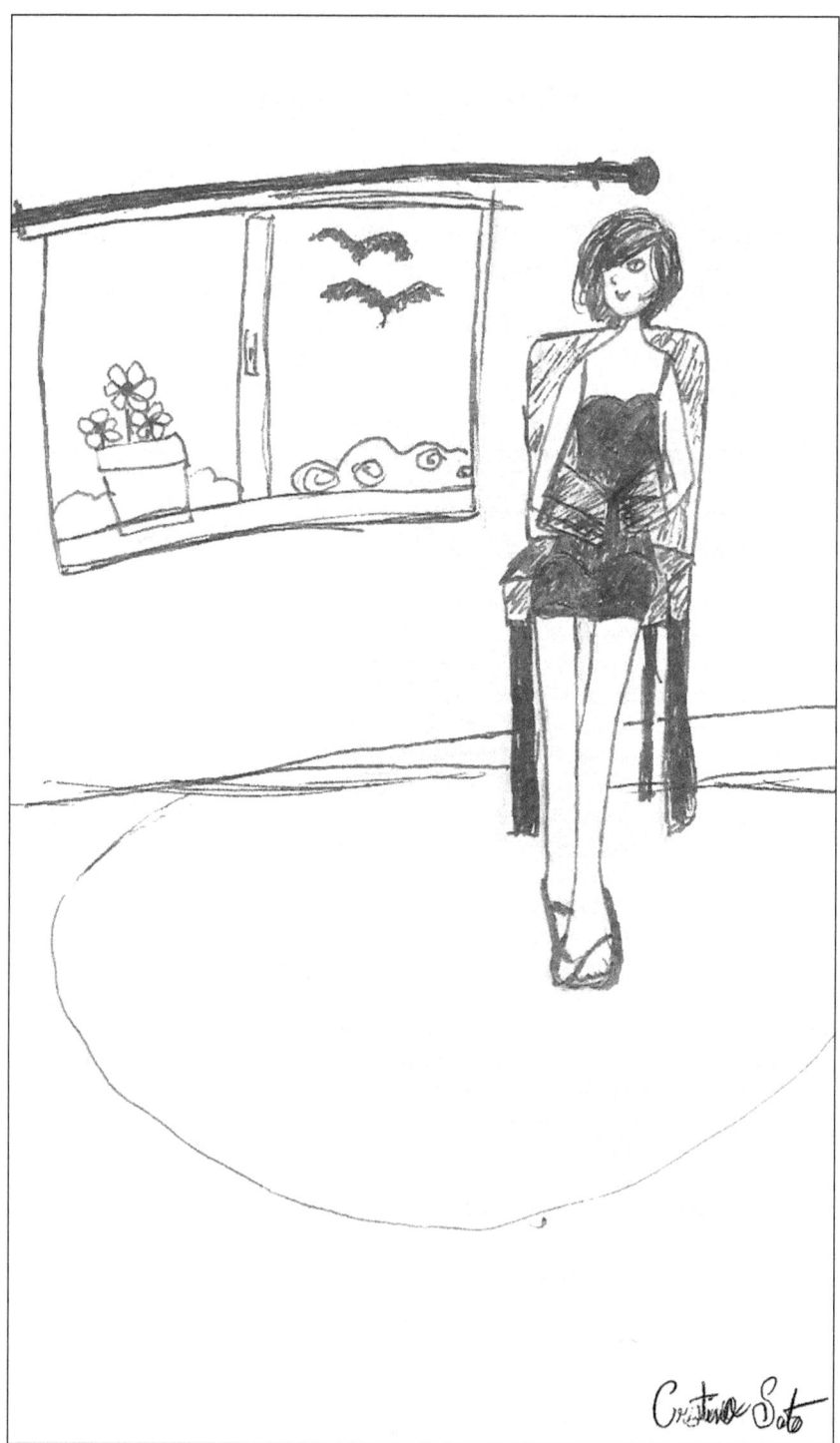

Idle Time

You may not think of your treatment time or convalescent time as idle time. I think of idle time as time that is not designated to a chore or a duty. Here we are having to take time to care for ourselves. There is nothing we absolutely need to do right now! Gee, what a concept.

Take this wonderful time, being home, to renew our acquaintance with our surroundings. How do they look? Do they reflect who you are today? Is there anything you'd like to change? Does it look too cluttered or too stark?

Sit in any of the rooms in your home and just look around. Is there anything you'd like to change? Use your imagination, be creative. Perhaps the pictures on your walls have been hanging there for a decade. Do you still enjoy looking at them or maybe a change is in order. Need a new bedspread? What about a new lamp? It doesn't need to take a lot of money. I've found many bargains shopping online. This may not be the right time for shopping, so try just imagining what new item would brighten up this or that corner. When you've gotten your strength back, then you can put your creativity into action.

Right now I just want to say, this idle time can be a fun time to plan for things that will give you pleasure when you've regained your energy.

Affirmation: *"My idle time is magical."*

Quote: *"Make your house a home."*

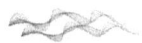

Scripture: *To get wisdom is to love oneself, to keep understanding is to prosper.*
                                            Proverbs 19:8

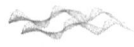

Idle Time

My Space For Thoughts, Reminders, Aha's

This space is for you to give gratitude, vent annoyances, remark on profound realizations, give appreciation to yourself, etc. Please use this area for whatever thoughts and feelings give you pleasure.

<u>Be sure to date each entry</u>. I find it fun to look back at things I've written months or years ago and think, "I said what??? When was that???"

_____

_____

_____

_____

_____

_____

_____

_____

Cancer Again?!

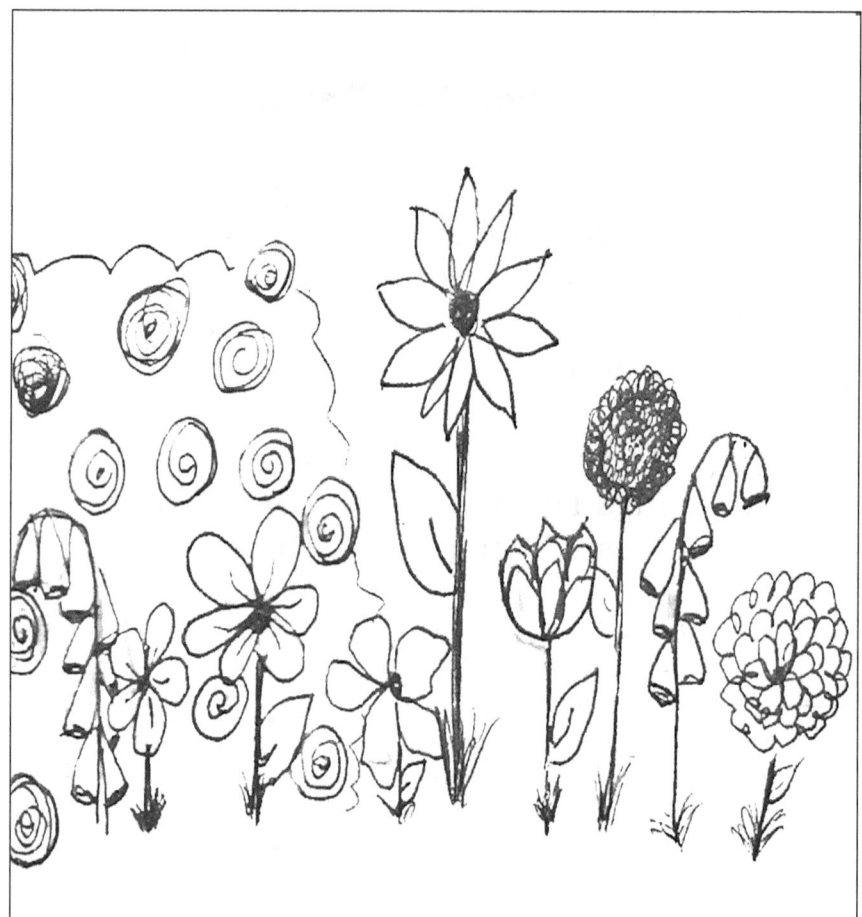

Humility

Humility: *the quality of being humble; modest sense of one's own significance.*

Yes, I've been forced to become humble during these two cancer experiences. What else could I do with people touching and probing around my body. It was important for me to always keep in mind, "It's all for my own good." But, I must say it's not always easy. You've got the little paper shirt and the little paper blanket, that are meant to cover you, but the paper slips and slides in all directions. Just thinking about it makes me feel humble.

I remember back when I was in third grade learning about the pilgrims. I was in a play and played the part of Humility. At the time, I had no idea of what that word meant. I do know the meaning now . . . loud and clear. Webster defines it as "modest sense of one's own significance". It's difficult to remain modest when you're exposed to exams, x-rays, etc.

Let's always remember pride is the alternative. Always stay in high opinion of your own dignity and importance. Always keep your self-respect and self-esteem.

The main thing is to be proud to be a survivor. Know you made the right choice in your treatment and care.

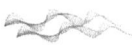

Affirmation: *"I am proud to be me."*

Quote: *"At times you'll wander off the path, just remember to get back on it."*

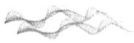

Scripture: *For the fear of the Lord is wisdom and discipline, fidelity and humility are his delight.*

Sirach 1-27

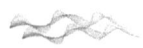

My Space For Thoughts, Reminders, Aha's

This space is for you to give gratitude, vent annoyances, remark on profound realizations, give appreciation to yourself, etc. Please use this area for whatever thoughts and feelings give you pleasure.

<u>Be sure to date each entry</u>. I find it fun to look back at things I've written months or years ago and think, "I said what??? When was that???"

_____

_____

_____

_____

_____

_____

_____

_____

_____

Cancer Again?!

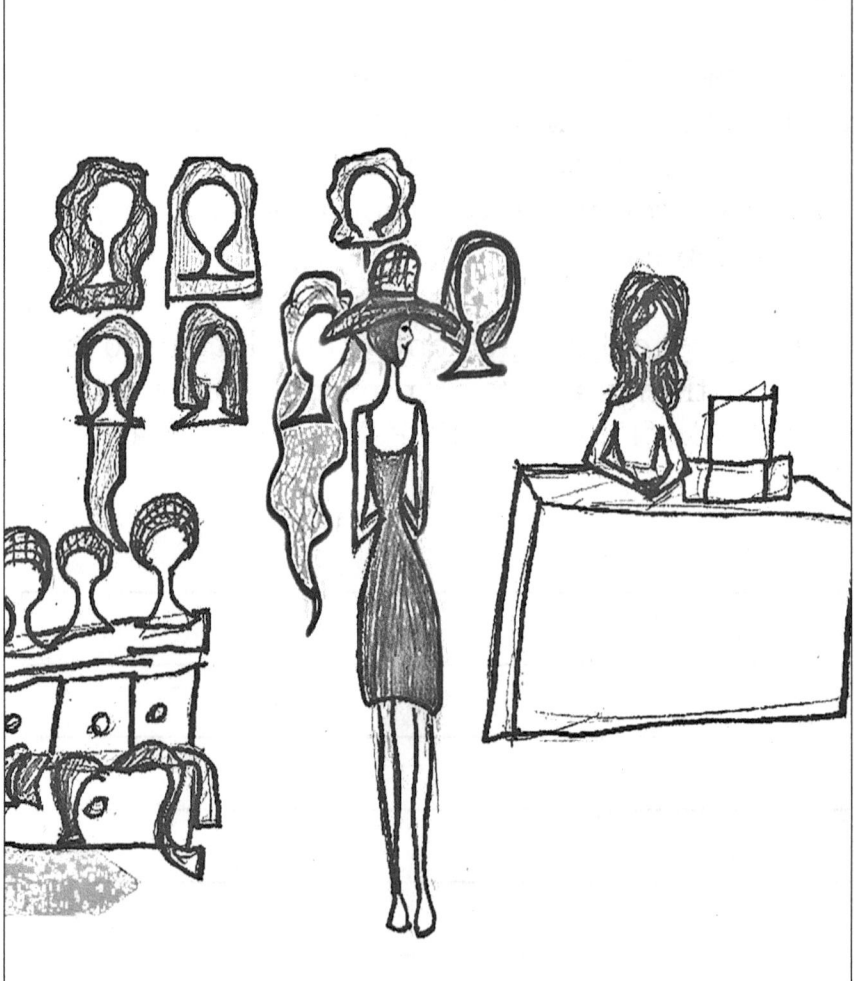

Hair or No Hair,
It Really Doesn't Matter

The first time I had cancer and was told I was going to be having chemotherapy, I didn't realize how devastating it was going to be to lose my hair. Being a woman, hair is a big part of my self-acceptance.

If you're dissatisfied with your hair now, too wavy, too curly, too straight, believe me you'll absolutely love your hair when you don't have any. About a week after my first chemo treatment, I was in the shower and started to wash my hair. It came out in handfuls, I just stood there and cried uncontrollably.

The voice inside me kept saying, "Take control, don't let the cancer control you." So I made up my mind to go and get a buzz cut, which left it about an inch all over. That was very freeing. My husband was so supportive he asked if it would help me if he also got a buzz cut? I declined his offer, but it was a very loving gesture. After the buzz cut my hair came out gradually giving me time to decide how I was going to go out in public? Bald or covered up? Well, vanity set in and I wore scarves and hats and always put on more eye makeup than I had worn before. Let me say, I'm not an overly vain person. I know I'm not beautiful, but I just want to look as good as I can, probably more for myself than for other people.

Your friends and family will always love you–with or without hair.

When my hair started growing in, it was such a welcome sight. And, the funny thing is, it came in curly. Curly little ringlets. My hair before chemo was straight. I was always using rollers, curling irons, etc. With the new curls it was simply wash and wear. As I remember after a few haircuts the curls disappeared. That was okay, I had hair and that's all that mattered.

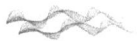

Affirmation: *"I am beautiful, just the way I am."*

Quote: *"Your hair does not define who you are."*

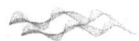

Scripture: *. . . For God loves nothing so much as the person who lives with wisdom.*
                                        Wisdom 7:28

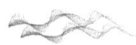

My Space For Thoughts, Reminders, Aha's

This space is for you to give gratitude, vent annoyances, remark on profound realizations, give appreciation to yourself, etc. Please use this area for whatever thoughts and feelings give you pleasure.

Be sure to date each entry. I find it fun to look back at things I've written months or years ago and think, "I said what??? When was that???"

_____

_____

_____

_____

_____

_____

_____

_____

_____

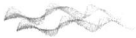

"My experience of Sandy when she was going thru her cancer diagnosis and chemotherapy is as a strong, determined woman making decisions, and moving forward with courage and faith. She retained her sense of humor and kept a positive attitude throughout."
Laurie Mann

Cancer Again?!

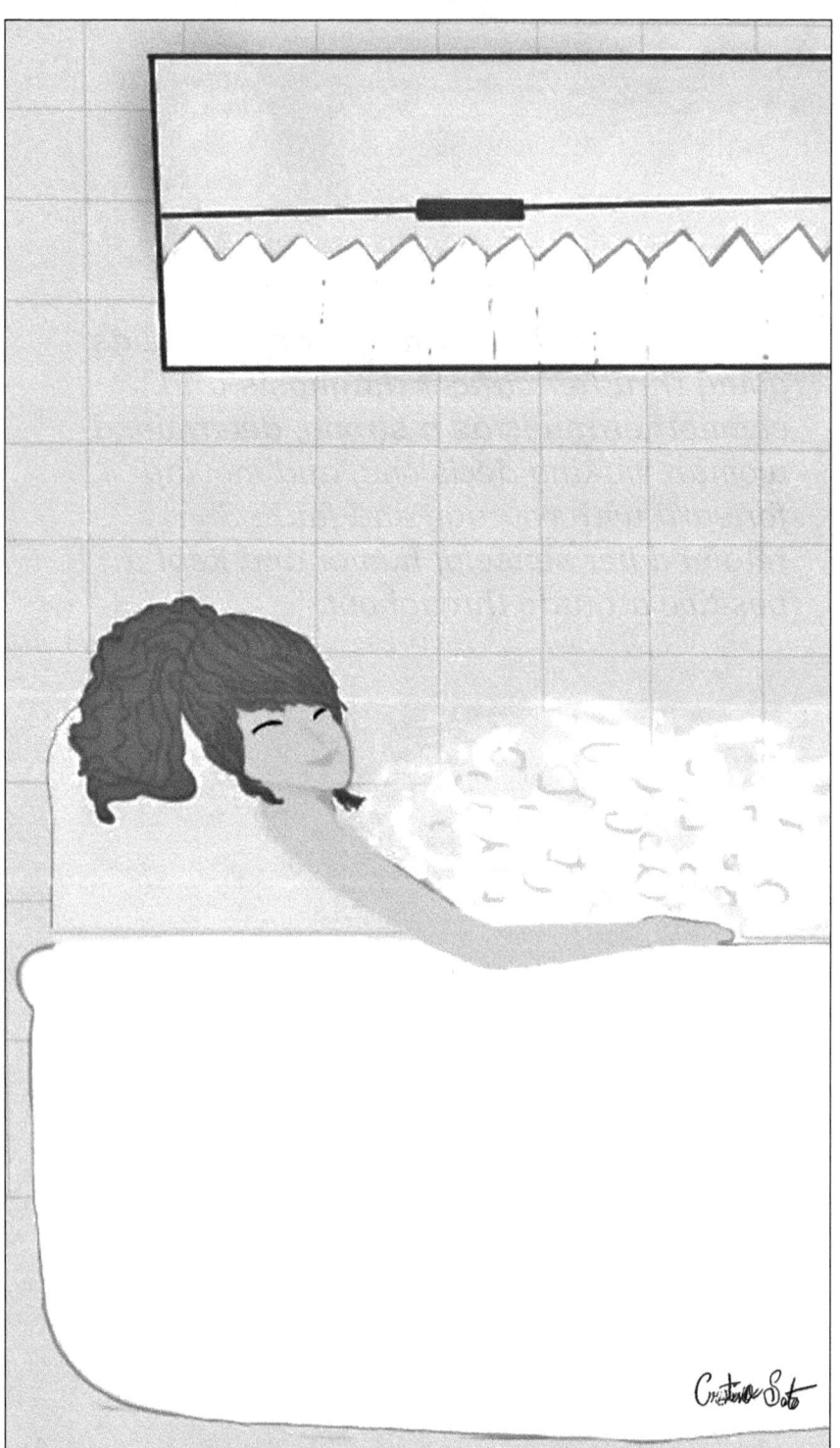

Comfort

If you are the type of person who always puts others first, now is the time to put YOURSELF first. Ask yourself, "How would I describe comfort?." Is it taking afternoon naps? Is it snuggling down with a good book, reading a little, dozing a little, mmmm, doesn't that sound good? Comfort may be being in the company of a good friend; sitting close and having a pleasant conversation.

Perhaps comfort to you is taking a stroll with nature, finding a pleasant place to sit, taking in the fresh, crisp air. How about going to the seashore and watching the waves? Or, maybe you see comfort as being home with your special pet. Feel the warmth of that body and know they can only give you unconditional love. I'd call that comfort.

Slipping my feet into my cozy slippers gives me comfort. A cup of hot chocolate also gives me comfort. And, a long leisure bubble bath gives me comfort.

My homework for you today is to write a list

of things that give you comfort, then move into action and bring about those things. Whether or not you're going through the challenges of cancer, always remember to give yourself some special time. Honor yourself. Make yourself comfortable. I promise it will lift your spirits and help your healing.

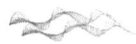

Affirmation: *"I listen to my body and comfort it."*

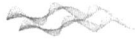

Quote: *"Ah! There's nothing like staying home for real comfort."*

Jane Austen

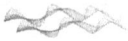

Scripture: *...because you, Lord, have helped me and comforted me.*

Psalms 86:17

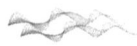

My Space For Thoughts, Reminders, Aha's

This space is for you to give gratitude, vent annoyances, remark on profound realizations, give appreciation to yourself, etc. Please use this area for whatever thoughts and feelings give you pleasure.

<u>Be sure to date each entry</u>. I find it fun to look back at things I've written months or years ago and think, "I said what??? When was that???"

_____

_____

_____

_____

_____

_____

_____

_____

_____

_____

Cancer Again?!

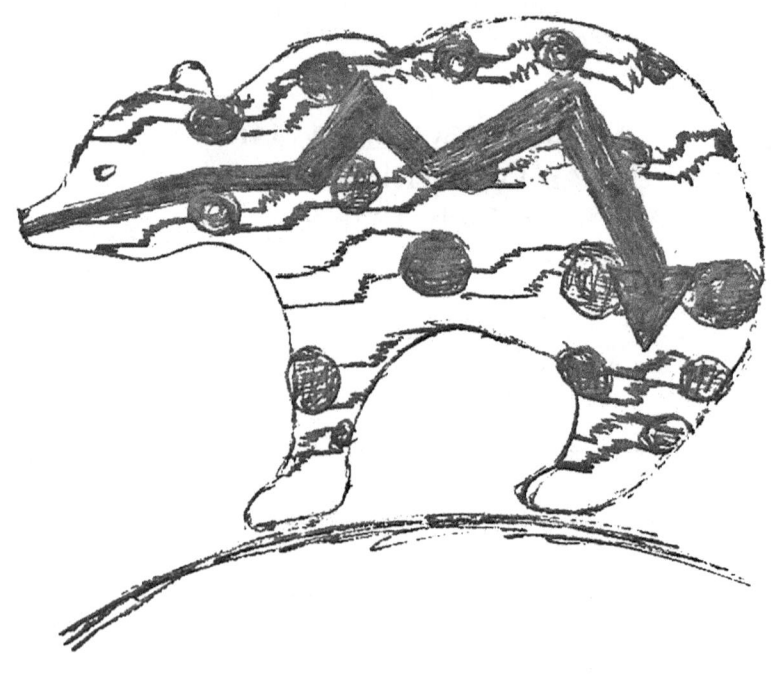

Inner Spirit

Please take a minute to settle in, sit quietly in a serene and quiet setting. Take a couple nice deep breaths. Sit in the silence for a couple of minutes. Let go of worries, your physical condition, any thoughts at all, *just be*.

Now ask yourself, "What is my inner spirit telling me?" Your inner spirit is where you will find your strength. It is where you will find your determination to move beyond your cancer. Know that cancer is just a blip in your being. Know that cancer does not define who you are. Know that cancer is your "wake up" call.

Sit quietly and listen to what your inner spirit is telling you. Your inner spirit knows that you are a perfect child of God. What is Spirit/God telling you?

As a cancer patient, *be* an example to others with your positive attitude. Show others that you will move beyond this circumstance and come out of it much stronger, and with a lot more awareness of who you are. Be the example of fortitude.

When you end this time of listening and talking with your inner spirit, move about the rest of you day with assurance that all is right in your world. Know that things will get better. Remember to be the example of strength and positive thinking.

Sometimes I think of my cancer as my wake-up call that made me understand and acknowledge my strength. As a two-time survivor, I want to reach out to others and let them know that everything is in divine order. I would love to sit in the silence with you and be strong for you; *know* that you will be strong for others.

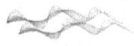

Affirmation: *"I am a perfect child of God."*

Quote: *"Sit in the silence, and know that your life has purpose."*

Scripture: *Do you hear the secret of God? And limit wisdom to yourself?*

Job 15:8

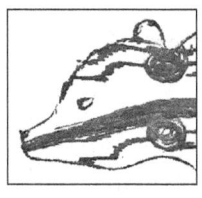

Appreciating Our Inner Powers

One night, Chief Clawing Bear was protecting the border of his village when he saw something glowing in the distance. As he started to walk towards it, he saw it was a plant. The Chief had to make his decision to either let the plant be or to investigate it more. This left him in a quandary but he made the decision to investigate it more.

When he touched the plant he gained special strength that no other human could have. He accepted his power and decided to protect his and neighboring villages with his new power, but first he was going to participate in the annual strength competition. There were three divisions. He made it to the last division when he lost his powers and lost the competition.

He was about to go back to his hut and feel sorry for himself, then he realized he needed to appreciate himself–powers or no powers. Chief Clawing Bear understood that his powers came from within himself, not from the plant.

By Joshua Soto, Age 10

My Space For Thoughts, Reminders, Aha's

This space is for you to give gratitude, vent annoyances, remark on profound realizations, give appreciation to yourself, etc. Please use this area for whatever thoughts and feelings give you pleasure.

<u>Be sure to date each entry</u>. I find it fun to look back at things I've written months or years ago and think, "I said what??? When was that???"

_____

_____

_____

_____

_____

_____

_____

_____

_____

_____

Cancer Again?!

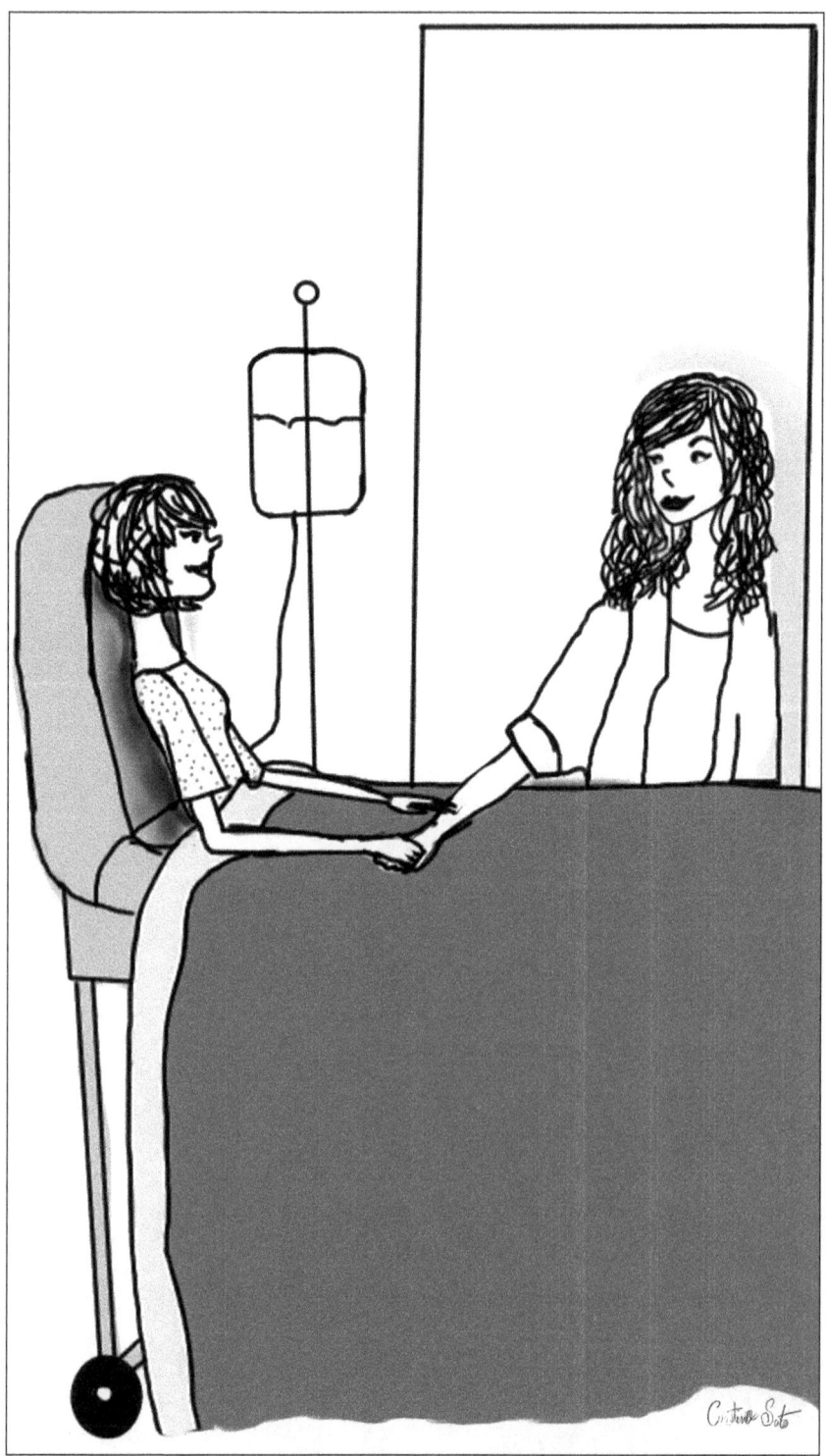

Support

Who is your support system? Do you have one? May I suggest you get one? You may want to just stay in bed and pull the covers over your head, but please don't do that. Reach out to others. Do you know you'll be giving them a gift? Yes, really! Family, friends and even strangers will want to help and support you in any way they can. You just need to ask.

I have friends who came and sat with me for three or four hours during my chemo treatments. What a blessing! We talked and talked; it took my mind off of that ugly poison they were pumping into my body. Yuk!

At first while sitting in the chair with the tube in my arm the nurses would offer me cookies, crackers and juice, and I would decline. Oh, I didn't want to be a bother to them; I knew they were very busy. But once I got the hang of it, I realized they were there to support me and they truly wanted me to be comfortable. And the cookies and juice took my mind off the chemo drugs. And I'd think, boy, this is a treat, I'm being waited on and getting good stuff to eat. Bring it on!

Then during my radiation treatments that were five-days-a-week and a 40-minute drive from my home, some friends would ask to drive me. I was capable of driving myself, but I thought, okay, it will make them feel better knowing they are helping me. It was a "win, win" for both of us.

Also, there are probably cancer support groups near you. Those groups are great ways to receive support and to offer support. If you don't find one nearby, how about starting a cancer support group yourself. It's a nice way to make new friends and be able to share your experiences.

Affirmation: *"I support others in their need and they support me."*

Quote: *"Always be willing to accept support and always be willing to offer support. It's a two-way street."*

Scripture: *How very good and pleasant it is when kindred live together in unity.*

Psalms 133:1

My Space For Thoughts, Reminders, Aha's

This space is for you to give gratitude, vent annoyances, remark on profound realizations, give appreciation to yourself, etc. Please use this area for whatever thoughts and feelings give you pleasure.

<u>Be sure to date each entry</u>. I find it fun to look back at things I've written months or years ago and think, "I said what??? When was that???"

_____

_____

_____

_____

_____

_____

_____

_____

Cancer Again?!

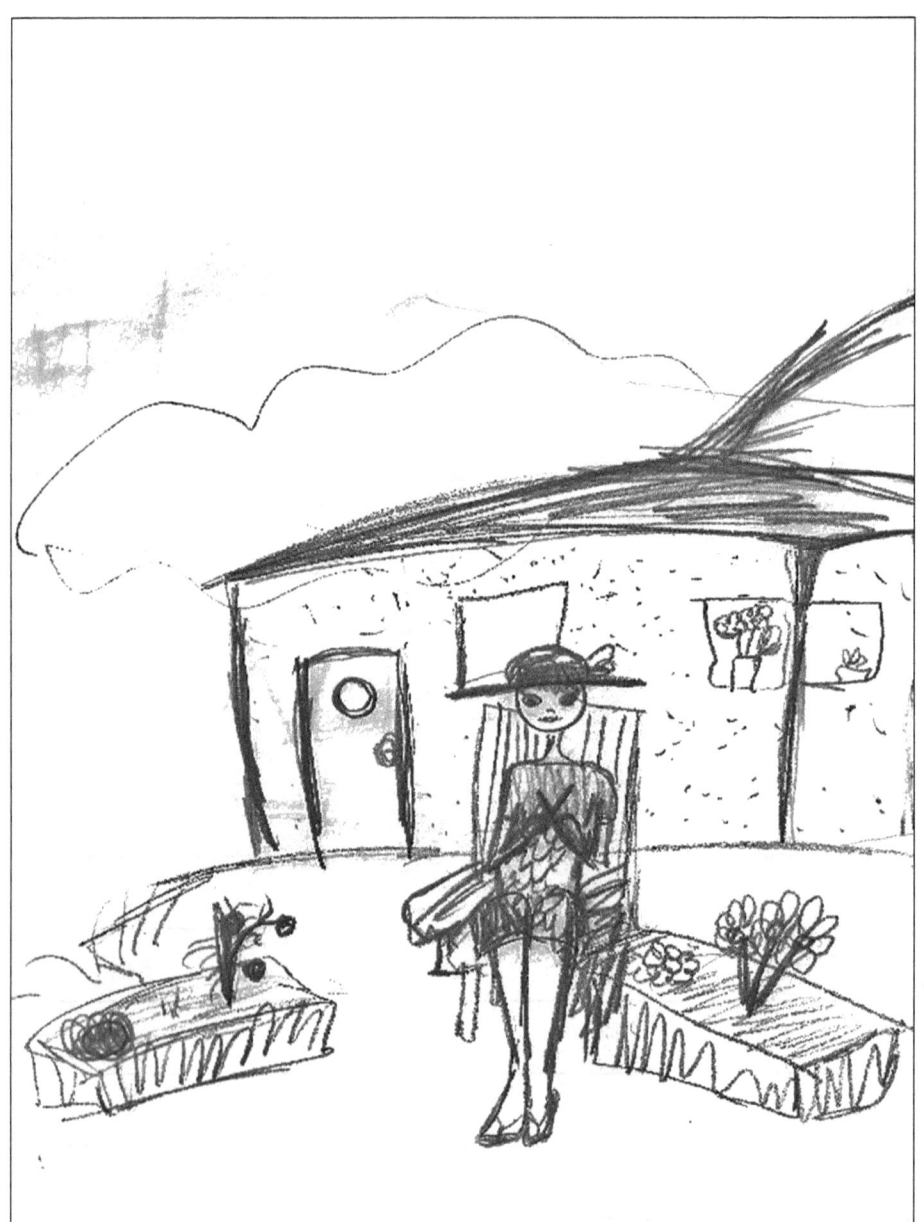

Take Time for Yourself

Just because you've been diagnosed with cancer doesn't mean your whole life now has to be all about your cancer. Even with the discomforts of the treatments, take time strictly for yourself. Be sure to get the rest you need. If you have children to tend to, ask a family member or a friend to care for them a short time during the day and then just treat yourself to time exclusively for yourself.

Lay down with a good book or read through your favorite magazine. Or, watch a simple, delightful sitcom on television. This is your time to comfort yourself.

Perhaps write a short note to a friend. Or, a thank you note to someone who has gone out of their way to be of assistance to you during this challenging time.

What about taking up a new hobby or craft. Learning something new will definitely take your mind off of you. Learn to knit, learn to sew, put together a model airplane. We all need a respite from worrying about the outcome of our tests, and our next treatment. Move yourself into the wonderment of something new. Something that gives you pleasure.

Did you know that preemie wards in hospitals need little, tiny hats for those very small premature babies? Start knitting little hats for those tiny infants. It's a blessing for them and you'll be doing a service. What better way to be creative and fill a need while you are getting through your health challenge experience?

Affirmation: *"I am a blessing to myself and others."*

Quote: *"Be good to yourself, love yourself."*

Scripture: *He maketh me to lie down in green pastures: he leadeth me beside the still waters. He restoreth by soul.*

Psalms 23:2-3

Take Time for Yourself

My Space For Thoughts, Reminders, Aha's

This space is for you to give gratitude, vent annoyances, remark on profound realizations, give appreciation to yourself, etc. Please use this area for whatever thoughts and feelings give you pleasure.

<u>Be sure to date each entry</u>. I find it fun to look back at things I've written months or years ago and think, "I said what??? When was that???"

_____

_____

_____

_____

_____

_____

_____

_____

_____

Cancer Again?!

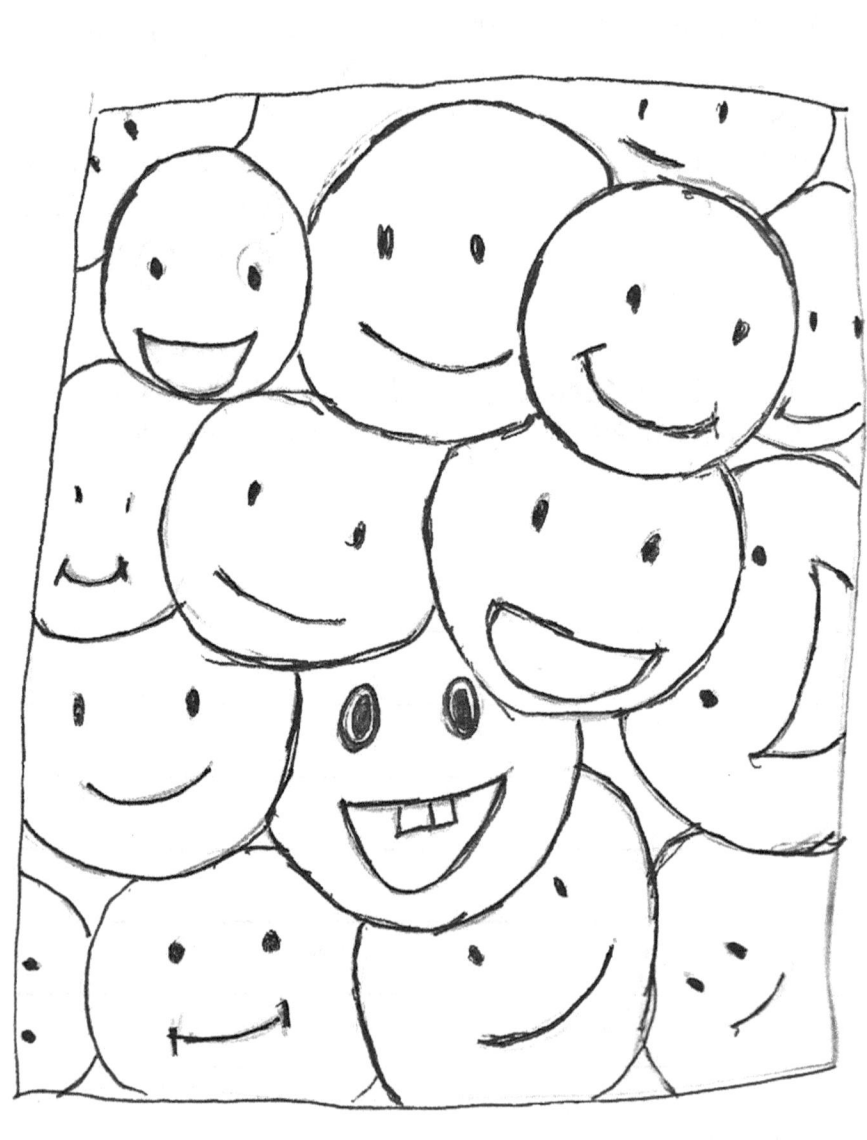

Cristina Sato

Let's Stay Positive

You've probably heard the saying, "Mind over matter?" How about let's change it to "Mind over body?" Now is the time to continue or try out prayer and meditation. Let's stay positive with laughter and support time with family and friends.

I like to sit quietly enjoying aromatherapy. Pick a scent you especially like and get it in a candle, spray or essential oil. The fragrance will help you to feel calm and help you to relax. I like rosemary and lavender. What is your preference? While you are sitting with these lovely scents, repeat a positive affirmation, something like, "My body is whole and well right now."

Another way to keep your spirits up is to have a massage or try reflexology (which is the stimulation of certain points in your feet.) Have you ever tried Reiki treatments? It rebalances your body's energy without being touched by someone.

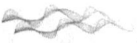

Affirmation: *"I am a unique and priceless person."*

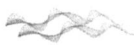

Quote: *"But what if I fail of my purpose here? It is but to keep the nerves at strain, to dry one's eyes and laugh at the fall, and baffled, get up and begin again."*
Robert Browning

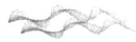

Scripture: *Finally, brothers, whatever is true, whatever is honorable, whatever is lovely, whatever is pure, whatever is commendable, if there is any excellence, if there is anything worthy of praise, think about these things.*
Philippians 4:8

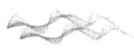

My Space For Thoughts, Reminders, Aha's

This space is for you to give gratitude, vent annoyances, remark on profound realizations, give appreciation to yourself, etc. Please use this area for whatever thoughts and feelings give you pleasure.

<u>Be sure to date each entry</u>. I find it fun to look back at things I've written months or years ago and think, "I said what??? When was that???"

_____

_____

_____

_____

_____

_____

_____

_____

_____

Cancer Again?!

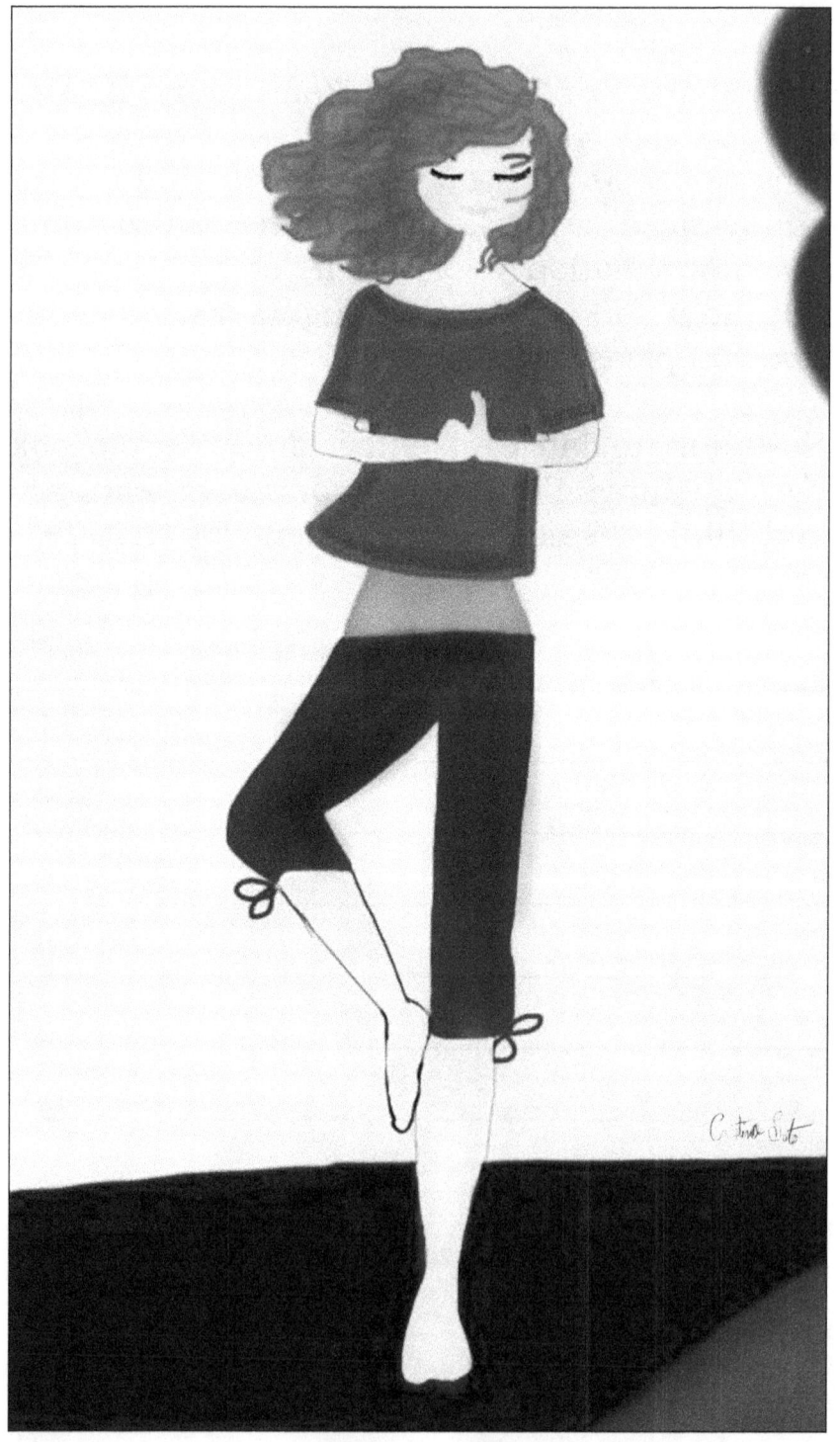

Inspiration

What inspires you? Have you ever asked yourself that question? That question causes me to pause and think . . . what inspires me?

Nature is one thing that inspires me. Nature causes me to believe in God. I think about dirt and things that grow out of the dirt, the plants and trees, and I think about animals, insects, fish, and birds. The air, the sun, the wind, and the rain nourishes every living thing including you and me. Only God could create what nature gives to us. That inspires me.

Perhaps you feel inspired by sitting quietly in a church or sanctuary, or watching a beautiful sunset. Or, you may be inspired by a particular author or composer. I find the poet, Rumi, inspiring. Who inspires you?

Now is the time to spend quiet moments taking pleasure from whatever or whomever inspires you. Give yourself that gift. Once you know what it is, let it wash over you and fill every cell of your body.

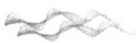

Affirmation: *"I hold what inspires me close to my heart."*

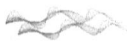

Quote: *"There are voices which we hear in solitude, but they grow faint and inaudible as we enter into the world."*
                                    Ralph Waldo Emerson

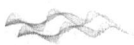

Scripture: . . . *The fruit of the spirit is love, joy, peace, patience, kindness, generosity, faithfulness, gentleness, and self control.*
                                    Galatians 5:22-23

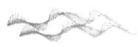

My Space For Thoughts, Reminders, Aha's

This space is for you to give gratitude, vent annoyances, remark on profound realizations, give appreciation to yourself, etc. Please use this area for whatever thoughts and feelings give you pleasure.

<u>Be sure to date each entry</u>. I find it fun to look back at things I've written months or years ago and think, "I said what??? When was that???"

_____

_____

_____

_____

_____

_____

_____

_____

Cancer Again?!

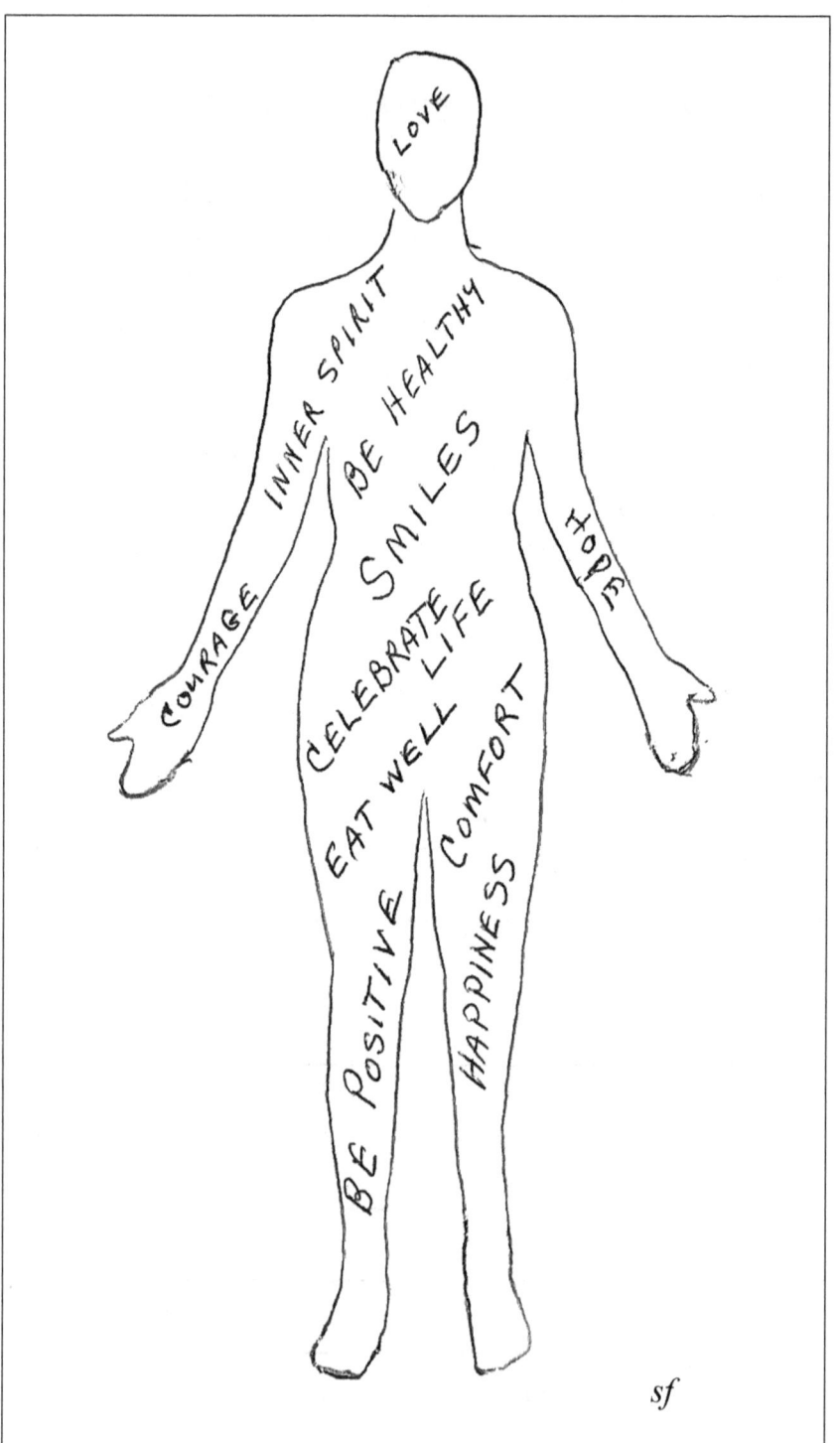

The Human Body

Have you ever sat quietly and contemplated the working of your body?

There are 300 different cell types in the human body. The average human body has 60,000 miles of blood vessels through which the heart pumps blood, and approximately 300 million capillaries.

All day, all night, all the time–the heart pumps blood throughout your body. Your blood carries oxygen and nutrients that your organs need to work.

Our bones protect certain parts of our body, our skull protects our brain, the spinal column protects the spinal cord and nerves, our ribs protect our heart, lungs and liver.

Think of all your moving joints–206 bones are in an adult human body.

Our skin is the body's biggest organ, it covers and protects everything inside our bodies. Can you imagine all the things that are happening in your body right now? To name a few, our skin cells are forming, our heart is sending nourishment throughout our bodies, our hair is growing, our toenails and fingernails are growing, our lungs are allowing us to inhale and exhale, our joints are allowing us to move every part of our body.

Our skin keeps us warm or cool. Our digestive system breaks down our food into a liquefied mixture. The digestive system allows the body to absorb nutrients.

All this is going on inside our bodies and we don't have to do anything. Our bodies are miracles. As I moved through my cancer treatments I became more and more awed by how my body renewed itself.

Every day now I thank my body for repairing itself and serving me. In my appreciation, I am eating healthy and exercising.

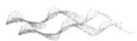

Affirmation: *"I am thankful for my strong, healthy body."*

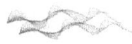

Quote: *"Who said chocolate is bad for you? If it raises your spirit, EAT IT!"*

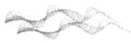

Scripture: *There is one body and one Spirit, just as you were called to the one hope of your calling, one Lord, one faith, one baptism, one God, and Father of all, who is above all and through all and in all.*

Ephesians 4:4-6

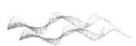

My Space For Thoughts, Reminders, Aha's

This space is for you to give gratitude, vent annoyances, remark on profound realizations, give appreciation to yourself, etc. Please use this area for whatever thoughts and feelings give you pleasure.

<u>Be sure to date each entry</u>. I find it fun to look back at things I've written months or years ago and think, "I said what??? When was that???"

_____

_____

_____

_____

_____

_____

_____

_____

_____

Cancer Again?!

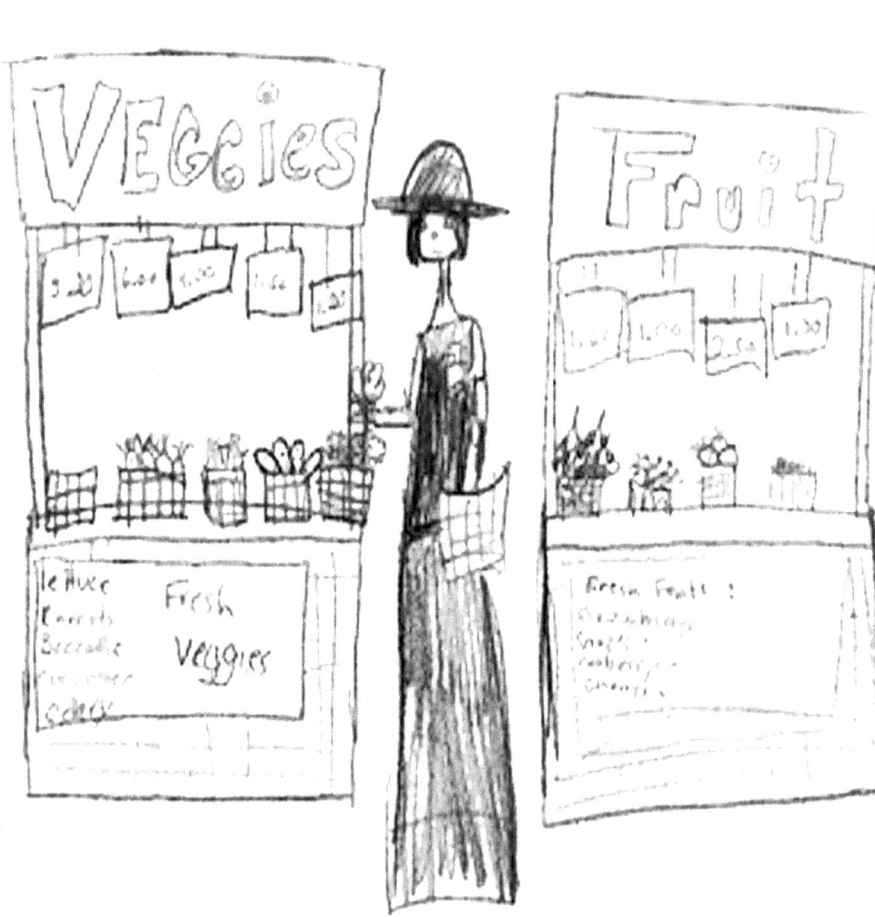

Eat Well and Live Well

Eat well and live well, and encourage others to do the same. Here is a quick list of some cancer fighting foods:

- Vegetables (broccoli, yellow squash, carrots, sweet potatoes, kale, spinach, swiss chard, brussel sprouts, bok choy, cabbage, cauliflower)
- Beans
- Onions and garlic
- Fruit (apples, apricots, bananas, cantaloupes, cherries, oranges, dates, figs, grapefruit, grapes, guava, honeydew melons, kiwi, lemons, limes, lychees, mangoes, nectarines, papaya, peaches, pears, persimmons, pineapples, plums, prunes, raisins, tangerines, watermelon, blueberries, raspberries, strawberries)
- Fish
- Tomatoes
- Mushrooms
- Almonds and ground flax seeds, peanuts and peanut butter
- Green tea

Remember, eating healthy keeps you strong, and helps your body rebuild tissue that has been damaged by treatment.

Affirmation: *"I am healthy and have tons of energy."*

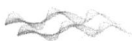

Quote: *"If someone gives you lemons—make lemonade or a lemon meringue pie would be nice."*

Scripture: *Whether therefore ye eat, or drink, or whatsoever ye do, do all to the glory of God.*

1 Corinthians 10:31

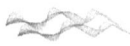

My Space For Thoughts, Reminders, Aha's

This space is for you to give gratitude, vent annoyances, remark on profound realizations, give appreciation to yourself, etc. Please use this area for whatever thoughts and feelings give you pleasure.

<u>Be sure to date each entry</u>. I find it fun to look back at things I've written months or years ago and think, "I said what??? When was that???"

_____

_____

_____

_____

_____

_____

_____

_____

_____

_____

Cancer Again?!

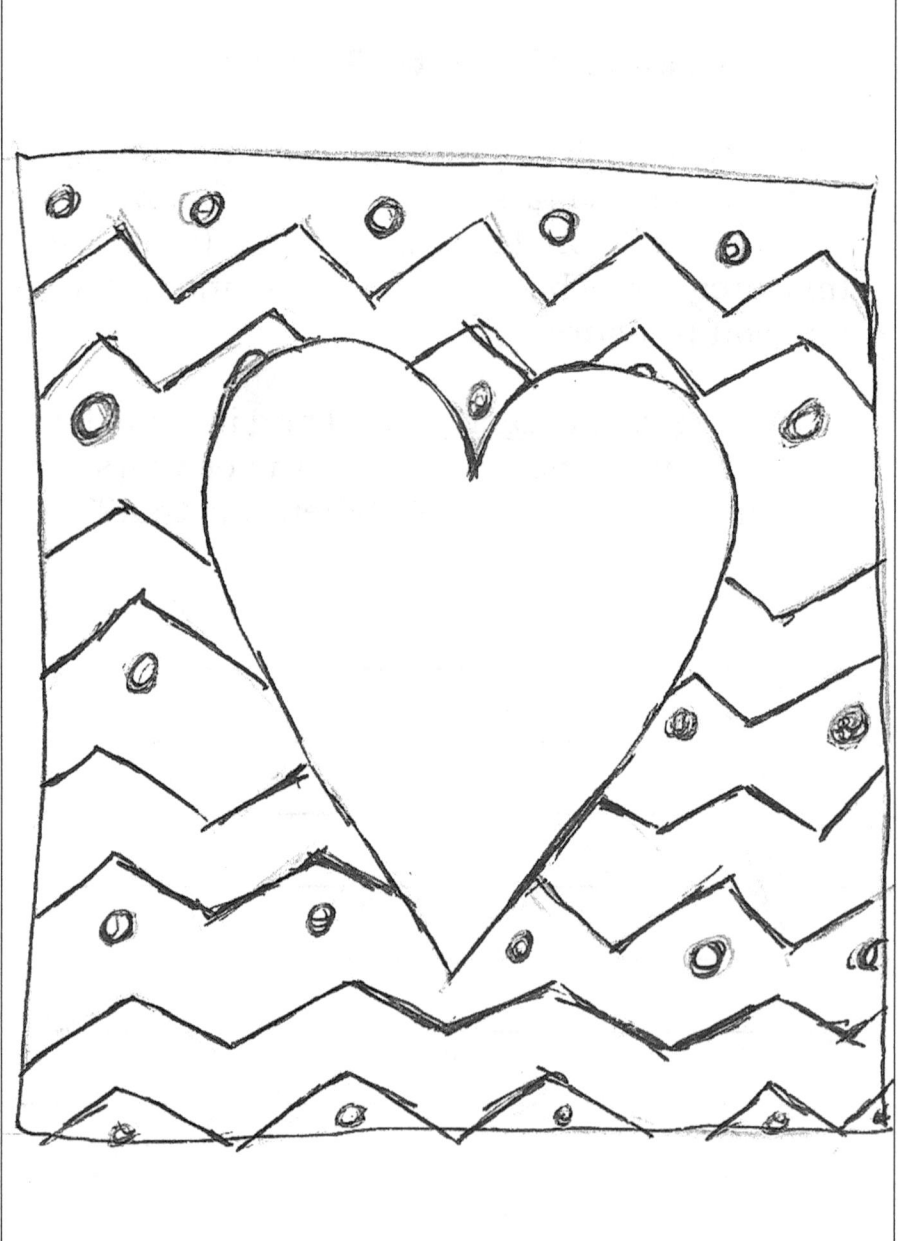

Love Yourself
Now is the Time

"It's all about me!" Yes. Perhaps through your life you haven't made yourself your first priority. Now is the time! If you are a mother, wife, grandmother, sister, daughter, auntie, BFF, please make yourself your first priority. It is fine to love and care for others, but at this particular time, please <u>put yourself first</u>. Now is the time to love yourself. Now is the time to appreciate yourself.

I listened attentively to everything the surgeon said and everything the oncologist said. I did exactly as I was told, I figured they are the experts. They are the ones with the degrees spending years to learn how to treat me. Yes, believe that. They went to school to learn how to treat YOU. So, pay attention to them.

When I was diagnosed with breast cancer in 2005, the surgeon told me he was going to do a lumpectomy and remove the cancer so no further treatment should be necessary. I left his office feeling okay. Thinking that is doable. But when I went to my first visit with the oncologist, he had another story. He started telling me about chemotherapy and radiation treatments. I said, "Oh, no, the surgeon said after removing the lump I shouldn't need further treatment." The oncologist said, "He's the surgeon, I'm the cancer specialist." With that, he turned on his computer and said, "Here are the facts. This is your cancer and this is the treatment for your cancer." There were no if's, or but's about it. I knew at that point I could have said, "No, I'll find an alternative treatment." But, why? He had the facts. Remember, he's the one with the medical degree, not me.

So, this brings us back to loving yourself. Put yourself first. Get yourself the best treatment possible.

Love Yourself

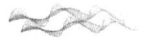

Affirmation: *"My body is healthy, strong and resilient."*

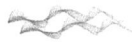

Quote: *"Yesterday I was clever, so I wanted to change the world. Today I am wise, so I am changing myself."*

Rumi

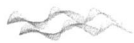

Scripture: *He getteth wisdom loveth his own soul: he that keepeth understanding shall find good.*

Proverbs 19:8

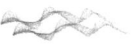

My Space For Thoughts, Reminders, Aha's

This space is for you to give gratitude, vent annoyances, remark on profound realizations, give appreciation to yourself, etc. Please use this area for whatever thoughts and feelings give you pleasure.

<u>Be sure to date each entry</u>. I find it fun to look back at things I've written months or years ago and think, "I said what??? When was that???"

_____
_____
_____
_____
_____
_____
_____
_____
_____

Cancer Again?!

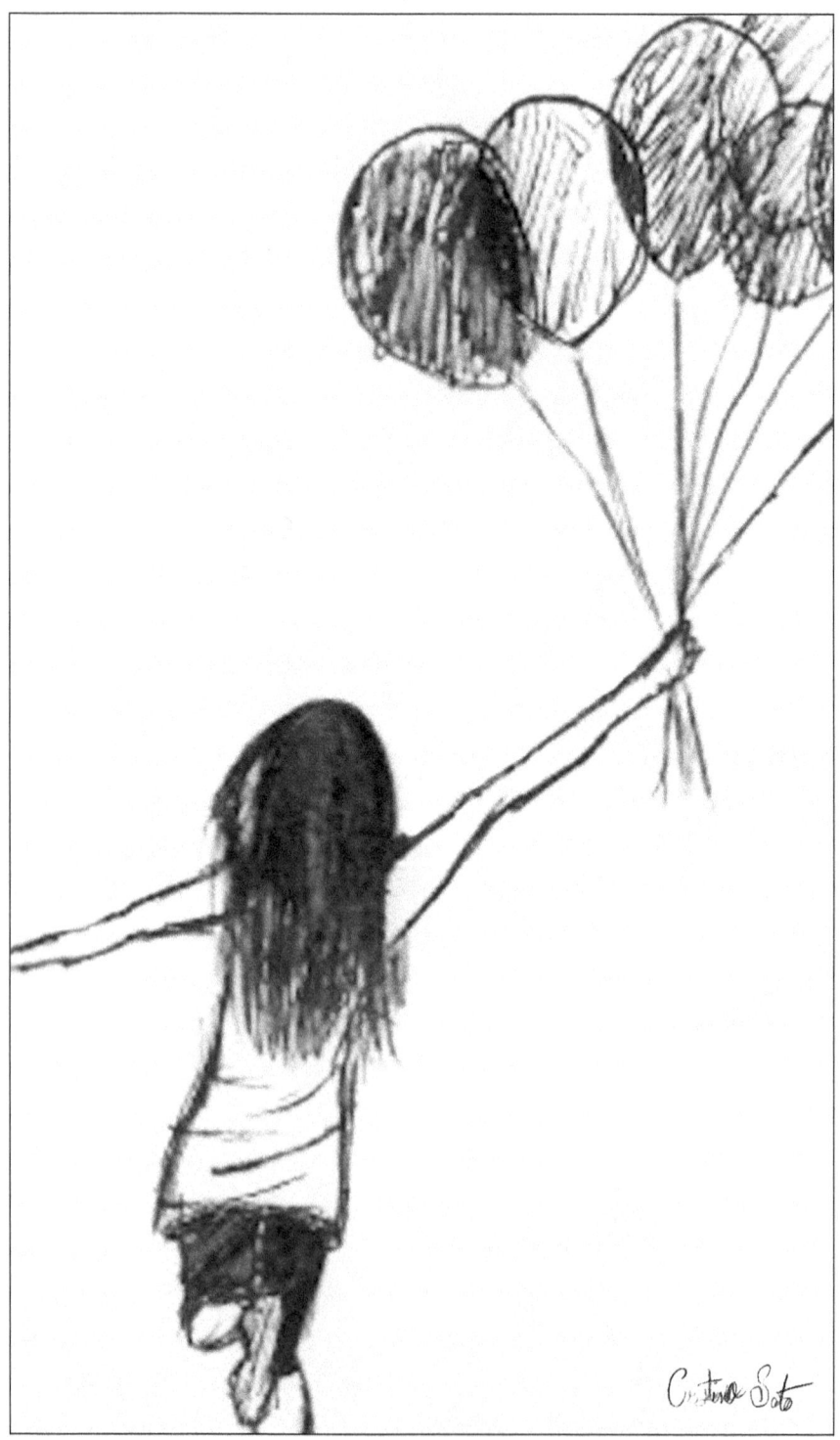

Celebrate Life

Keep giving yourself gifts. We all like gifts. Or, how about a "treat"? My 6-year-old granddaughter defines a "treat" as an "unexpected pleasure". After she gave me that definition, every day I try to give myself or give someone a "treat".

A treat might be an excursion to someplace you haven't been in awhile or some place you've always wanted to go. Plan to take some friends along–they will all want to celebrate with you.

Another fun treat might be to have a party when you have completed your treatments. Celebrate Life! Ask guests to bring a cancer fighting food dish along with the recipe. Give the party a food theme and have "best recipe", "most creative", "most colorful", "healthiest" awards. This will educate your guests and get them involved.

Shopping is another way to celebrate. Treat yourself to a new outfit or a new pair of shoes, or keep it simple with a pretty scarf or necklace. YOU are special, my beloved sister–you deserve to be treated that way!

Someone told me a fun thing to do would be to have a gift for yourself on the days you have your chemo treatments. When you hear you'll be having the treatments, take a day and buy yourself 4 or 6 gifts (however many treatments you're scheduled to have), wrap them in pretty paper and open one on a treatment day. If you'd rather be surprised with your gifts ask someone else to shop for you. I didn't do that when I was going through my treatments, but I wish I had. It sounds like fun and a great way to celebrate life.

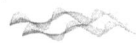

Affirmation: *"I am special."*

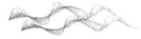

Quote: *"Love is the energy of life."*
Robert Browning

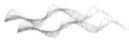

Scripture: *Thou wilt show me the path of life; in Thy presence is fullness of joy: at Thy right hand there are pleasures for evermore.*
Psalms 16:11

My Space For Thoughts, Reminders, Aha's

This space is for you to give gratitude, vent annoyances, remark on profound realizations, give appreciation to yourself, etc. Please use this area for whatever thoughts and feelings give you pleasure.

<u>Be sure to date each entry</u>. I find it fun to look back at things I've written months or years ago and think, "I said what??? When was that???"

_____

_____

_____

_____

_____

_____

_____

_____

_____

Afterword

Sandy Foreman is an incredible person. For over 30 years, I have watched her *make* things happen. When the doctor told her she had cancer, her response was "How do we make this go away?" Her oncologist set a strategy of surgery, chemotherapy and radiation, which she followed knowing that afterwards the cancer would be gone. During her treatments, she would take a day for chemotherapy and then be right back to her daily life.

The most discouraging thing was the loss of her hair. Sandy is not a vain person but she does take pride in here appearance. So during this time, she played with different ways to present her head using scarves, hats and wigs; to finally being OK with just going places bald. And when her hair started growing back, coming out in little curls, it was actually fun for her. She is a true example of "If someone gives you lemons, make lemonade."

The second time, though disappointing, her attitude was "I've done this once so I can do it again and I know I will be OK." Even though the surgery and treatments were more severe she made it an exciting adventure. This time the doctor said that she was a good candidate for robotic surgery. During the surgery, the mechanism sparked and punctured a vein. The puncture was easily repaired without any residual effects. Afterward, she named the *daVinci*® Surgical Systems' robot "Sparky". Her recovery room was on the 10th floor of the Queens Medical Center in Honolulu. She refers to her stay as being at a resort with an ocean view. Again, she makes lemonade.

I have felt the love that she exudes. I am blessed, living, and sharing my life with such a remarkable person. Since we married, over thirty years ago, she has been my spiritual and inspirational guide.

Charles Foreman

Purchasing Information

Special terms: order direct from the publisher if you have an organization interested in purchasing quantities of *Cancer Again?!* for fundraising, please contact:

Russ Ranch Productions
P.O. Box 517
Woodacre, CA 94973-0517 USA
email: survr2x@aol.com

Also available for purchase online and from your local bookstore.

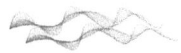

www.ingramcontent.com/pod-product-compliance
Lightning Source LLC
Chambersburg PA
CBHW071716040426
42446CB00011B/2088